MW00928105

WHY

REIKI

WORKS.

Why Reiki Works.

Series "Why Alternative Medicine Works"
By: Sherry Lee
Version 1.1 ~July 2022
Published by Sherry Lee at KDP
Copyright ©2022 by Sherry Lee. All rights reserved.

No part of this publication may be reproduced, distributed or transmitted in any form or by any means including photocopying, recording or other electronic or mechanical methods or by any information storage or retrieval system without the prior written permission of the publishers, except in the case of very brief quotations embodied in critical reviews and certain other noncommercial uses permitted by copyright law.

All rights reserved, including the right of reproduction in whole or in part in any form.

All information in this book has been carefully researched and checked for factual accuracy. However, the author and publisher make no warranty, express or implied, that the information contained herein is appropriate for every individual, situation, or purpose and assume no responsibility for errors or omissions.

The reader assumes the risk and full responsibility for all actions. The author will not be held responsible for any loss or damage, whether consequential, incidental, special, or otherwise, that may result from the information presented in this book.

All images are free for use or purchased from stock photo sites or royalty-free for commercial use. I have relied on my own observations as well as many different sources for this book, and I have done my best to check facts and give credit where it is due. In the event that any material is used without proper permission, please contact me so that the oversight can be corrected.

The information provided in this book is for informational purposes only and is not intended to be a source of advice or credit analysis with respect to the material presented. The information and/or documents contained in this book do not constitute legal or financial advice and should never be used without first consulting with a financial professional to determine what may be best for your individual needs.

The publisher and the author do not make any guarantee or other promise as to any results that may be obtained from using the content of this book. You should never make any investment decision without first consulting with your own financial advisor and conducting your own research and due diligence. To the maximum extent permitted by law, the publisher and the author disclaim any and all liability in the event any information, commentary, analysis, opinions, advice and/or recommendations contained in this book prove to be inaccurate, incomplete or unreliable, or result in any investment or other losses.

Content contained or made available through this book is not intended to and does not constitute legal advice or investment advice and no attorney-client relationship is formed. The publisher and the author are providing this book and its contents on an "as is" basis. Your use of the information in this book is at your own risk.

2

Table Of Contents

Introduction.

Are you interested in the title: Why Reiki works? The purpose is not to intrigue but to inspire and persuade you that the power of Reiki resides within you.

Reiki is beneficial energy that gives joy and illumination to the lives of everyone who embrace it. It is an energy that can accomplish life's petty goals. Often, the way Reiki operates appears magical.

According to Reiki, the world is energy vibrating at various frequencies. Thought and action are both composed of energy. Every object in the physical universe consists of energy vibrating at various frequencies.

Since energy cannot be destroyed, it remains in its current state until it is transformed into other forms or through chemical reactions to generate new energy vortices. Reiki provides you the ability to transform the bad into the positive.

Reiki is a healing technique and a way for spiritual growth. However, Reiki's energy is neither good nor negative by itself. It corrects bad energy and improves positive energy flow. It eliminates blockages, increases energy levels, and revitalizes everything sluggish and unhealthy.

Some meditations are taught during the Reiki initiation process. People who have meditated in the past would find it simple to reach the ideal condition following Reiki initiation.

Those new to meditation will discover they can enter the meditative state with minimal ascetic practice. In addition, their relationship with God and the universe would be quietly transformed, and they would be able to relate profoundly to living and nonliving objects.

Consistent practice of Reiki to heal oneself and others will result in clearer mental processes, improved memory, and increased overall energy. The essential demand made by the energy is that we submit to its intellectual power and permit it to direct us to our desired aims.

Reiki is not confined to medical clinics and examination tables. It can become a part of your daily life and enrich it beyond your wildest imagination! It is not dark magic or witchcraft. It is proof that the universe is abundant and that all we have to do is to realize our desire to focus our energy and tap into the wealth.

Let's get started.

Chapter 1: What Reiki Is and How It Works.

Reiki is a supplemental therapy that can facilitate healing. Reiki is the vital energy that permeates all living things. The stresses of daily life cause blockages and imbalances within the body.

Since Reiki covers all levels of existence, it creates the conditions for unification and equilibrium on all levels of the individual. Reiki facilitates restoring physical, mental, emotional, and spiritual balance to optimize health and healing.

A Reiki practice or treatment is a simple technique that allows your body to "align" through palm-to-palm contact with the practitioner. Reiki is risk-free and can be experienced as a heightened sense of oneness and harmony. Reiki practitioners assist individuals in attaining a more unified state of health.

Reiki improves conscious health and awareness. It is a complementary healing modality and a collaborative process between the client, the practitioner, and the universe.

How does it work?

Reiki is multidimensional as it provides the environment for healing the source of a problem at its origin's physical, mental, emotional, or spiritual level. Reiki attunes the individual to his or her natural state of equilibrium. Balance creates the conditions for health and healing to take place.

The Reiki practitioner does nothing to the recipient; rather, he or she allows Reiki to be present for realignment and rebalancing. Self-healing is the only form of healing. The individual's natural healing mechanisms are activated when the environment is optimized. Reiki is a non-invasive practice. Therefore, Reiki is completely safe and has no adverse side effects.

Reiki is not a religion; you are not required to believe anything to learn and practice it. It is not dependent on belief and will function whether or not you believe in it. Neither is it required to be directed by a practitioner. Reiki is not a replacement for medical and other health care procedures but can complement, support, and improve them.

Reiki is utilized in many hospitals across the world. It is applied during surgery, in the emergency room, oncology, pediatrics, neonatology, labor & delivery, and rehabilitation departments. Advantages include:

* Reduces pain.

* Reduces anxiety and encourages relaxation.

* Helps the body eliminate harmful poisons.

* Controls the energy flow throughout the body.

* Provides solace and tranquility to the terminally ill.

* Encourages health and well-being.

* Improves and speeds the body's natural healing processes.

Reiki is taught, and pupils receive "attunements" directly from a licensed Reiki Master (Teacher). It is taught in three sequential levels known as degrees, each consisting of varying lengths and durations of workshops.

First Degree Reiki is utilized for self-healing and administering Reiki to another physically present individual. Reiki of the Second Degree is utilized when the recipient is at a distance. Third Degree Reiki is the Master Level, intended for people who wish to teach Reiki exclusively.

Although many healthcare professionals can be Reiki practitioners, no special experience or certifications are required to learn Reiki. Reiki practitioners are often trained in supplementary techniques such as acupuncture, massage, herbal treatments, and yoga.

You might inquire with practitioners of these approaches, wellness or holistic health facilities, or health food stores in your area. You can also conduct a network or an online search via word of mouth.

You will seek a practitioner who utilizes Reiki consistently for self-healing and has been attuned to at least First Degree Reiki by a Reiki Master.

The practice of Reiki isn't a religion.

* Reiki is not a replacement for seeking or getting medical care.

* Reiki is not a replacement for effective, necessary, and recommended medicine.

Reiki is a safe supplemental treatment that, combined with conventional and alternative healing methods, can help your health and healing. It is utilized in many hospitals and has no adverse effects.

Chapter 2: Five Major Advantages Of Reiki.

Everyone has heard of Reiki or "Universal Life Energy." It is a well-known spiritual practice that utilizes natural energy to treat physical diseases and alleviate challenging life circumstances.

Dr. Mikao Usui increased awareness of this treatment method. Although no scientific evidence supports the existence of such a global life force, people who practice or receive reiki healing techniques have never been let down. Now let's examine the top five benefits of Reiki:

Not only will Reiki offer stability to your life but also to the lives of others around you. Often, I have observed that reiki healers are surrounded by such positive energy that their sheer presence may fix challenging problems.

Reiki masters must undergo significant alterations to improve their healing powers. Dr. Mikao Usui outlined five rules that reiki healers must adhere to maintain high healing skills. Below are the five reiki principles:

• Just For Today: I will count my blessings.

• Just For Today: I will not be angry.

• Just For Today: I will not be anxious.

• I Just For Today: will be truthful.

• Just For Today: I will be kind to all living things.

Those who adhere to these ideas religiously achieve inner peace and can connect with the universe's beneficial energy.

We have all heard that reiki assists in the healing of physical ailments but how many of us are aware that Reiki can also be used to resolve any problem? With the aid of Reiki, intention manifestation is achievable. You can anticipate miracles from these treatment methods.

I have employed a combination of reiki and Feng Shui, Reiki and the laws of attraction, and Reiki and angel communication to attain my goals. Whether or not you believe it, Reiki can solve any problem.

Reiki serves the ultimate good of all, which means it doesn't harm. Suppose you are in a difficult scenario, such as a disagreement with your supervisor. If you apply Reiki to this issue, it will work out for both of your highest good. This suggests that all concerns will be handled, or fantastic job chances will separate you.

It improves intuitive capabilities. Reiki will often advise you when you are caught in a difficult position and cannot decide what to do. Sometimes you can sense what will occur. Reiki will prevent you from taking incorrect action.

It is beneficial for healing pets. Even animals respond favorably to a reiki treatment. Reiki is a calming and uplifting energy that assists in reducing physical pain and discomfort, especially in animals whose souls are pure.

Chapter 3: Why Your Life Needs Reiki.

You have probably been performing Reiki therapy your entire life without your knowledge. What do you do when you are hurting? You reach out and grasp the aching portion of yourself. This is Reiki.

It entails seeking pain relief by channeling energy into the affected location. Anytime you get injured as a child, your mother would likely touch and kiss the affected area. This is the purest kind of Reiki therapy.

Love and healing. What could make a person feel better than that?

Reiki is all about utilizing the energy surrounding us to aid in healing our pains, aches, diseases, emotional, physical, and mental problems, and disorders. Imagine if you could apply this same healing energy to every aspect of your life. Well, my friend, you can!

Reiki is a natural and risk-free approach that anybody can utilize for self-improvement and spiritual healing. It has been proven helpful against every illness and ailment and always produces a positive effect. In addition, it acts in tandem with all other medical or therapeutic methods to alleviate side effects and improve healing.

Our bodies consist of trillions of vibrating, energetically active cells. We are energy! I recently read that if you compressed all the non-energy components of our body, they would equal the size of a sugar cube.

The rest of our body is composed of pure energy. Therefore, it stands to reason that when we suffer from a sickness, physical or otherwise, it is likely due to a blockage in the normal flow of energy that constantly flows in and out of our body.

We consist of 99 percent energy!

According to scientific evidence, all living and nonliving things are composed of energy. I propose the well-known author and microbiologist Dr. Bruce Lipton's book, Biology of Belief.

Okay, so we are almost entirely energy. How do we correct energy blockages that influence our feelings, actions, and lives? Here is where Reiki comes into play. Energy is required to resolve energy-related issues.

Reiki is based on ancient wisdom lost for millennia before being rediscovered in Japan approximately one hundred years ago. This path is referred to as Reiki (Japanese for Rei, which means Universal or Sacred and Ki which means Life Force) and the seven chakras or primary points through which healing energy flows in our body.

If your energy flow is disrupted, you may experience disease, illness, aches, pain, headaches, despair, or other responses. Your body is indicating that something is wrong and must be fixed. An energetic obstruction must be eliminated. Because you are predominantly energy, energy is the most likely solution to these issues.

Are you unsure of an unseen energy flow?

It is normal to be dubious of something you cannot observe, correct? What are your thoughts on radio waves? TV signals? What's Internet? Microwaves? Wi-Fi? Smartphones? We do not see unseen waves that make these technologies that most of us cannot live without, yet we are willing to accept them. Why? Because we know their efficacy.

Reiki shows its efficacy daily in homes, businesses, hospitals, farms, and gardens. It is highly recognized by the medical community, with over 900 hospitals in the United States offering Reiki as a complementary therapy.

However, Reiki is not an alternative method. Doctors and other health care professionals advocate and practice conventional medicine because, although they may not fully comprehend how it works, they know it does.

Reiki, the Soft Treatment.

Reiki is a gentle, relaxing therapy that alleviates stress, headaches, and pains. It can also be useful in assisting individuals with emotional and mental health issues such as depression, anxiety, stress, and frustration, and the rigors of cancer treatment, heart surgery, post-traumatic stress disorder, and other debilitating conditions. As stated previously, it is increasingly utilized in clinics and hospitals.

Vitality and Your Body.

Harold Saxon Burr, a Yale University School of Medicine researcher in the 1920s, proposed that diseases may be identified in the body's energy field before the onset of clinical symptoms. Using SQUID (Superconducting Quantum Interference Device) devices, scientists map how diseases modify the biomagnetic fields surrounding the body.

Using a SQUID magnetometer, Dr. John Zimmerman launched a series of significant experiments on therapeutic touch at the School Of Medicine, the University Of Colorado in Denver in the early 1980s. Zimmerman noticed that a TT practitioner's hands produced a massive pulsating bio-magnetic field. The frequency of the pulsations varies from 0.3 to 30 Hz (cycles per second), with most activity occurring between 7-8 Hz (Figure 2).

Hand bio-magnetic pulsations have a frequency that is similar to brain waves. According to scientific studies, the frequencies essential for healing spontaneously sweep back and forth through the whole spectrum of therapeutic frequencies, boosting healing in any part of the body.

Considering all these factors makes it clear why Reiki can be a vital part of your life. You might substantially reduce your medical expenses if you avoided clinics, hospitals, uninsured prescriptions, treatments, and procedures. Extending the practice of placing your hand on a sore spot to a complete session with a Reiki practitioner can lead to improved health and faster healing, resulting in lower costs.

Reiki practitioners always have your best interests in mind, but you must believe in Reiki's ability to help you heal or resolve a problem or circumstance. If you do not believe Reiki will help you, you are producing negative energy, which will undoubtedly impair the results of any Reiki treatment you receive.

Alternatively, if you feel Reiki may help you, your positive energy will be felt and contribute to your therapy's favorable outcome.

Caution: Don't expect miracles. Reiki practitioners cannot treat ailments overnight, much as physicians cannot (although occasionally it does seem to happen).

In addition to improving your health, Reiki can affect your life in different other ways. Let me offer you a few. Reiki is effective in healing pets and other animals, in gardens to improve yield, in business to encourage output and income, in relationships to assist in resolving issues you and a loved one are experiencing, and yes, even in preparing for final exams!

Chapter 4: Different Methods Of Utilizing Healing Reiki Energy.

There are almost infinite methods to use what you've learned and send healing Reiki energy to people, places, and circumstances in need. Here are ten outstanding beneficiaries of clever Reiki energy:

1. Utilize the healing Reiki energy to assist in the healing of your previous scars, difficulties, and blocks that are still present in your body. Everyone has them.

Who better than oneself to work on? You will become a stronger Reiki practitioner and be able to assist others more effectively. If you have completed the training for Reiki Level II and learned the sign for distant healing, you can also transmit Reiki energy to your past and future selves.

2. Animals - Animals enjoy receiving Reiki and often do not have the resistance to healing caused by people's egos.

3. Countries in need - You can send Reiki to the starving people in Africa, the entire continent if you choose, or even the entire planet. Send them a mass healing if there is a natural calamity or individuals in need. The world requires your services.

4. Send a small amount of Reiki into your food before consuming it. Use the Reiki power symbol if you are familiar with it; otherwise, simply place your hands over your food and desire for the Reiki to enter it immediately.

5. Use Reiki to cleanse your home in your house or business. It functions similarly to sage and other cleansing treatments. Also, if you enter a space with much negative or stagnant energy, place Reiki symbols in the four corners, and you will feel the negativity dissipate.

6. Job interviews or first dates - Send Reiki energy to the circumstance and yourself and the other individuals involved before an interview or first date. You will be surprised by how easy the actual scenario gets!

7. When something breaks down, such as your automobile, radio, or computer, transmit Reiki energy directly into it to restore its power.

8. Toward objectives or anything you intend to manifest. If you are familiar with the manifestation symbol, send it alongside the growth sign to accelerate the time required for your goals to become a reality.

9. Heal addictive behaviors in yourself and others - Use the mental/emotional symbol to assist in the healing of addictive behavior such as codependence, drug and alcohol issues, and smoking.

10. As a supplement to Western Medicine for different disorders - Since Reiki energy is compatible with practically all therapeutic modalities, it can be

used to treat physical ailments ranging from cancer to the common cold.

Although these are all wonderful individuals, locations, and circumstances to send Reiki healing energy, the possibilities are endless. I encourage you to apply your Reiki course skills in your unique way.

Chapter 5: How Reiki Harmonizes All Aspects Of Your Being.

Reiki is a natural energy that permeates the universe. You can focus this energy on different objectives, including spiritual growth and healing through initiation and training.

Reiki harmonizes the mental and emotional parts of your existence. It brings spiritual energy into harmony with your physical self. Reiki harmonizes all aspects of your being and complete being with the universe.

It cultivates your sense of oneness with the cosmos and lets you perceive life holistically in all its aspects and expressions. Reiki is utilized for self-healing, healing others, and connecting to metaphysical, spiritual energy via potent initiation rituals.

How can Reiki Help?

Reiki makes you aware of spiritual truth by allowing you to experience the warmth and vibration of high energy immediately. It broadens your cerebral, spiritual, and emotional pathways to heighten your spiritual sense. Reiki promotes spiritual development by enhancing insight during meditation. It is utilized to treat spiritual difficulties, emotional obstacles, and bodily ailments.

No, you do not need to "believe" in Reiki, but please unplug any "disbelief" as it drastically hinders comprehension. I'd like to question your worldview so that you might be liberated from any restrictive ideas.

I advise you to adopt a holistic approach to your personal and global health. Through the practice of Reiki, I aspire to generate profound insights into the nature of reality and the self. Please open your heart and mind for a once-in-a-lifetime Reiki encounter.

Reiki functions in the same manner that EVERYTHING does, following the laws of nature. No, not the scientific laws we learned in school but the natural laws that transcend traditional scientific theories.

The truth is that conventional views of human nature and the human being are extremely reductionist and limited. Our species has been reduced through material empiricism to atomistic electro-mechanical machines comprised of elements and chemicals smoldering within our bodies. When we increase our knowledge and consciousness, the concept of Reiki becomes pretty straightforward.

Reiki is easy to experience but exceedingly challenging to explain. Certainly, Reiki's protocols, techniques, and history are plain and simple to comprehend, but the subject of how Reiki works might be enigmatic and incomprehensible to rational, scientific intellect.

Sir James Jeans made a profound discovery in the 1920s that the universe appears more like a vast thought than a great machine. Many experiments conducted by physicists over the past 80 years have demonstrated this to be true.

From this perspective, the significance of universal connectivity and the power of consciousness increases tremendously. Thoughts of healing a person produce healing; thought influences thought, and since we are all thought, we impact everything! Presto!

Reiki heals on the spiritual, emotional, intellectual, and physical levels by changing blocked or negative energy patterns into positive, circulating energy. Remember that everything is energy, even mass. Fire is energy. Atoms and particles are sources of energy. Both positive and negative thoughts contain energy. Both love and hatred are forms of energy.

The physical human body is low-frequency vibrating energy. The conscious and spiritual aspects of humans vibrate at higher frequencies. The distinction between these occurrences is the frequency of vibration.

To suggest that some realms do not exist because we cannot see them is like claiming that a high frequency exceeding 20,000 Hertz doesn't exist because we cannot hear it. Remember that human intellect is hardly the final measure of the cosmos. More likely, the human intellect may be one of our greatest barriers to knowing the universe.

Thought influences matter just as the mind influences the body. Mental and spiritual energy with a high frequency may not be directly perceptible by our physical sense organs, but mental activity's repercussions present themselves in different bodily situations.

Many diseases, including headaches and ulcers, are physical manifestations of mental impulses. Smiles and laughing are also physical manifestations of healthy emotional energy.

When you comprehend oneself in this manner, it makes sense that Reiki can promote physical health gains. Reiki is compassionate energy comparable to the positive energy generated by meditation, love, or prayer, which vibrates at higher frequencies and brings about bodily changes.

Studies indicate that neighborhoods surrounding meditation centers have lower crime rates. Therefore, the influence of positive energy extends from the individual through the community to all of humanity.

Holistic Healing utilizing Reiki.

Most physical ailments are treated with chemical medications. When a student seeks Reiki therapy after years of stomach problems, back pain, or headaches, it is not surprising that one Reiki treatment can reveal that they were unknowingly storing bad energy such as fear, anger, or guilt. Negativity becomes lodged in the digestive organs, the muscles and the brain, preventing the natural flow of energy.

When the reason for a headache or ulcer is mental or emotional, no amount of medication will cure it. Medications may offer temporary comfort by masking or suppressing symptoms but rarely address the underlying causes of disease.

Why has the modern concept of the human body been reduced to chemical equations? Why don't we see ourselves in their entirety and address our health in terms of our entire being? This is the objective of Reiki and other holistic healing methods.

Amazingly, conventional science understands the world in terms of cause and effect due to the scientific method it employs and not because of the nature of reality!

Similarly, our perception method determines what we observe in a healing setting, whether allopathic or energetic. Chemical reactions are seen when a chemist experiments.

When a Reiki healer arranges healing, other hands, energetic responses are observed. So, which is genuine? Perhaps nothing is real until it is tried and experienced personally. This perspective is consistent with postmodern notions of multiple truths and quantum physics concepts.

Reiki healers channel healing energy by opening their minds and hearts. Reiki is directed via awareness to eliminate or alter disease-causing harmful or obstructed energies by laying one's hands on another learner. Reiki generates feelings of lightness, brightness, and compassion by enhancing harmony with the universe.

Chapter 6: What Is A Reiki Attunement?

In the 1980s, attunement became a common way to refer to a person's connection to universal energy. The dictionary definition of attunement is harmony or the sensation of being at one with another being.

Being in harmony with everything demands inner balance and a condition of receptivity. Therefore, to be receptive to the kind of energy known as Reiki, one must be in a state of receptivity, and Reiki cannot be forced on anyone.

The ground and all of nature - on land, water, and air — possess their energy. Whoever is attracted to a plant, animal, or bird for no apparent reason and is conscious of this connection is aware of that kind of nature's energy. Others, including herbalists, forest rangers, and farmers, are in sync with nature.

As we all learned in science class, energy cannot be created or destroyed but can change form; there are countless types of energy. One type of your energy is referred to in many languages as life force, qui, ki, prana, and many others.

Usui Reiki Ryoho is a spiritual practice that utilizes a unique kind of universal energy distinct from life force energy; hence, you must be initiated into this form of universal energy by a licensed Reiki Shihan (teacher).

While Mikao Usui's second awakening directly connected him to a potent type of universal energy, different people have connected/utilized other kinds of universal energy throughout history.

Each time you receive an initiation/empowerment/attunement from a Reiki Shihan (teacher), a shift occurs in your mind, body, or spirit as your connection to the universe becomes slightly more expansive, allowing more universal energy to flow through you. It would require years of study, discipline, and practice to fully open up to the universe, which is beyond human comprehension.

It took Mikao Usui years of accumulating diverse information to achieve even his initial awakening. After 3 years of diligent Zen practice, days of intense meditation, and hours of unconsciousness, he did not connect to universal energy until his second waking.

As common as the term Reiki attunement has become, it is sometimes forgotten that Usui Reiki Ryoho is a spiritual practice. The fact that attunement is merely the beginning occasionally among the missed.

Richard Rivard noted that Reiki Ryoho was used for all forms of hands-on therapy in Japan until the 1980s, which is why it is crucial to trace the lineage of a Reiki Shihan (teacher) back to Mikao Usui. The system created by Mikao Usui is unique, even though many teachers have integrated other techniques into the style they teach.

Usui Reiki Ryoho contains no deep, dark secrets; nonetheless, one qualified Reiki Shihan compared the institution Gakkai to the Freemasons in that no one knows what happens because members do not discuss matters outside their closed doors.

Even though no one outside of the Gakkai knows what Mikao Usui knew and did, the hours of instruction from the proper instructor can help you get the understanding to grow spiritually and improve all aspects of your life. Usui Reiki Ryoho produces healing as a byproduct; the Reiki energy balances and surrounds to promote health and happiness.

Reading an interview that Paul Mitchell, a teacher of Usui Shiki Ryoho (one of the styles of Usui Reiki Ryoho), gave in October 2003, I discovered a suitable approach to describe how a teacher initiates another into the spiritual practice of Usui Reiki Ryoho.

He said. "Initiation is the sacred rite passed down from master to master that enables us to access Dr. Usui's gift. It is a form of spiritual communication." I disagree with the use of Dr and master in front of Mikao Usui's name, but that doesn't diminish my admiration for the wisdom in Paul Mitchell's explanation of attunement.

Mikao Usui did not earn a degree; instead, he took a new road, leaving tracks in the sand that no tide can erase. He was a highly knowledgeable and wise individual who merited the title of Sensei, which translates as a revered teacher.

Many people like me have spent years learning, continue to learn and grow and consider it an honor to be selected as someone's instructor. You may also encounter someone who has passed multiple Reiki levels but doesn't mention Reiki.

It is not uncommon to see medical physicians and other professionals who have finished various levels of Usui Reiki in this century. Once you have been attuned to universal energy and taught to subdue your rational mind and ego, Reiki may flow into and enrich every positive aspect of your life.

You can feel many energies within yourself with direction and practice that are not universal and are therefore not Reiki. The Reiki energy form is distinct from all others, and a Reiki attunement cannot be defined in terms of other energy forms.

I have received what is often referred to as attunements in many Usui Reiki Ryoho forms. Consider universal energy, the pure water flowing from a spring in a pristine natural forest. The vibrations of universal energy's love and harmony are always the same, but the human through whom it flows can alter how the energy looks, feels, and smells.

The flavor of water sipped from a paper cup will differ from that from a glass or tin cup, depending on what other beverage was previously consumed in the cup or glass and how well it was cleaned. Likewise, universal energy flows through the body, mind, and spirit. Unaltered universal energy has a very fine, delicate texture that, for some of us, is accompanied by a delicate aroma.

It is left to the individual to decide what they wish to study, but not all paths lead to the same destination. Words have multiple meanings, which multiply when translated from another language. Do you know what Japan means? The kanji for Japan means "The origin of the sun" or "Land of the Rising sun

Chapter 7: What Is The Reiki Natural Healing System?

Universal life force energy is the meaning of the term reiki, where Reiki means universal, and ki means life force energy. Life force energy is the vital power that permits all living things to survive and reproduce.

It is a unique art in which the reiki practitioner channels this concentrated form of life force energy through their chakra system (invisible energy vortices in the human body). The reiki energy runs through the practitioner's crown chakra and to their palm chakra.

Reiki energy has a calming and relaxing quality; it is an excellent stress reliever. Within minutes of having treatment, most individuals fall asleep. The healing process is divinely led.

It has the intrinsic intelligence to comprehend and heal entirely. In other words, the healing energy already knows how and what to heal; we do not need to train it. Reiki energy is all-knowing and healing-capable.

Reiki healing techniques are rather straightforward and may be mastered with diligence. There are no prerequisite requirements for learning it. Reiki can be simply learned by anyone willing to study and has an open mind.

Attunement is the procedure by which the reiki master transfers healing power to the trainee. Typically, the process of attunement entails invoking angels, gods, and goddesses. After the attunement, the reiki student can properly channel energy and heal himself and others.

A typical Reiki session lasts one hour. The practitioner can feel the flow of Reiki energy through the body and convey this energy to the healed person. In Reiki, there are secret symbols that aid in the healing process. Reiki Remote Healing is also a possibility.

It is possible to send distant healing to someone who is not physically present with the reiki practitioner. Reiki distant healing is extremely effective and convenient for the healee, as they can receive it from the comfort of their own home.

There are seven primary chakras in the human body: Anahata (heart chakra), manipuraha (solar plexus), swadhistan (sacral plexus), Muladhara (root chakra), vishuddhi (throat chakra), ajna (third eye chakra) and Sahasrara (crown chakra) (crown chakra).

The proper functioning of these chakras is vital for the proper functioning of the human body. We can easily cure and restore health and well-being to all chakras and the body parts and organs associated with each chakra with the aid of Reiki.

Reiki is mostly utilized for positive thinking and goal realization. Reiki eliminates all negativity from the body, mind, and consciousness and assists in the emergence of positive thoughts. Many healing procedures in Reiki facilitate realizing one's objectives and ambitions

Chapter 8: The Crucial Symbols Used In Reiki Attunements and The Healing Process.

Reiki symbols are drawn from Sanskrit and are primarily influenced by this ancient language. To connect with "particular" healing frequencies, these symbols increase energy and help direct the flow of Ki (or chi in Chinese). A Reiki master teaches these symbols during the Second Degree of Reiki. These pictorial/written symbols are utilized in the attunement and healing processes.

The involved energy, Ki, was and remained the foundation of all of Chinese medicine, where it is called chi. Its name is a mantra that helps one connect with the symbol's energy; it means "Correct thought is the essence of existence" or "Correct consciousness is the source of all things."

During the Reiki attunement, the energy of the attunement leads the Reiki symbols to become a stimulus, and the specific energy represented by the symbol present during the attunement becomes the response.

During an attunement, you are given a connection to the energy via symbols, which are utilized to aid concentration. Cho Ku Rei, the first of the three symbols learned at Level 2 Reiki, is utilized to concentrate and protect energy. Sei Hei Ki and Hon Sha ze Sho Nen are the last two.

Utilize the first three Reiki symbols in concert with one another to customize the Reiki energy for each client. The first symbol, the power symbol, magnifies Reiki like a magnifying glass magnifies the sun's energy.

A Reiki master can deliver attunements to instruct someone in Reiki or provide someone with a deeper understanding of Reiki than is often encountered in treatments. For a Reiki channel to be properly attuned, authentic Reiki symbols are essential.

Reiki practitioners can become adept at using these symbols to heal themselves and others, locally and remotely, with the correct training. The Reiki practitioner facilitates the client's spiritual, mental, emotional, and physical healing by simply laying hands. When utilized to treat pain, the symbol might diminish the intensity of the pain and gradually cause it to disappear.

Sei Hei Ki Often referred to as "the Mental-Emotional Symbol," Sei Hei Ki aids in restoring mental-emotional equilibrium. The emblem of mental and emotional health balances the right and left hemispheres of the brain.

When feelings of fear, anxiety, wrath, or depression arise, you can utilize the sign on yourself (or others). Creating oneness with a portion of yourself that has suffered lays the groundwork for employing the mental/emotional symbol to bring gentle healing.

Their use does not necessitate meditation skills or years of spiritual practice. A great deal of practice employs the symbols to enhance energy, do distant healing, repair the subconscious mind, create an affirmation, and remove the atmosphere of negative energy. With practice, the significance of the reiki symbols will diminish, and the focus will shift to the "intent" of the precise energies required.

The Reiki practitioners do not believe in imparting their knowledge of Reiki and Reiki symbols to aspiring students who have not acquired particular Reiki levels. Numerous practitioners employ this symbol when administering treatment.

In any case, a substantial number of these more recent symbols exist and are employed by an increasing number of Western Reiki practitioners to augment their practice.

Typically, a Reiki instructor or master demonstrates the Reiki symbols and the necessary concepts for employing them to a student. These are sacred healing symbols that facilitate the circulation of Life Force Energy. These symbols facilitate connection with life's vital energy forces.

Chapter 9: Utilizing Reiki To Assist Surgery.

Reiki therapies would greatly assist those scheduled to have a medical operation, whether a simple or complex procedure. Certain surgical procedures are required to cure the body of certain disorders completely. Reiki would be of considerable assistance in these situations, although not immediately.

Reiki is the optimal complement to contemporary medicine. If your doctor informs you that you have uterine issues, you should not rely solely on a Reiki practitioner to treat you. Continue with your doctor's prescribed meds and procedures and seek the assistance of a Reiki practitioner to accelerate the healing process.

Therefore, Reiki can assist in two ways. It can make you feel better quickly and allow your physician to feel the Reiki energy within him to treat you more effectively. Reiki's distance healing enables any practitioner to send the appropriate energy to the doctor and all other medical personnel with whom you will interact. Full Reiki therapy yourself would also greatly assist during the surgical procedure.

Surgical procedures that use Reiki are reputed to be more efficient and successful. When Reiki is used for an estimated three-hour surgery session, the patient will likely spend only two hours in the operating room. Moreover, probably, the disease's consequences will also be resolved swiftly.

Reiki can also be utilized during the healing process. After surgery, patients typically experience pain. The pain a person experiences during the post-surgery recovery period can be alleviated by Reiki's ability to call forth energy, love, and healing. Consequently, the patient will be able to live a richer and more independent life in the coming days.

The experiences of surgical patients who received Reiki would further demonstrate that healing occurs simultaneously with necessary treatment. When most patients would need to transport medical devices such as dextrose and catheters home, those who had Reiki therapy sessions performed on them would leave the hospital with nothing but their clothing attached.

Reiki practitioners and recipients who will soon undergo medical surgery are advised to get at least fifteen full Reiki sessions before the surgery date. If the energy could be transmitted to the accompanying physician, surgeon and nurses, the effect would be even more profound.

Doing so can cut in half the time you need to recover. You will not have to wait six weeks on your recovery bed for the pain to lessen and the wounds to heal, thanks to Reiki. Within three weeks, you should be completely recovered, and you can use the remaining time to continue your self-improvement using Reiki concepts. Today, get well quickly and effectively.

Reiki therapies would greatly assist those scheduled to have a medical operation, whether a simple or complex procedure. Certain surgical procedures are required to cure the body of certain disorders completely. Reiki would be of considerable assistance in these situations, although not immediately.

Reiki is the optimal complement to contemporary medicine. If your doctor informs you that you have uterine issues, you should not rely solely on a Reiki practitioner to treat you. Continue with your doctor's prescribed meds and procedures and seek the assistance of a Reiki practitioner to accelerate the healing process.

Therefore, Reiki can assist in two ways. It can make you feel better quickly and allow your physician to feel the Reiki energy within him to treat you more effectively. Reiki's distance healing enables any practitioner to send the appropriate energy to the doctor and all other medical personnel with whom you will interact. Full Reiki therapy yourself would also greatly assist during the surgical procedure.

Surgical procedures that use Reiki are reputed to be more efficient and successful. When Reiki is used for an estimated three-hour surgery session, the patient will likely spend only two hours in the operating room. Moreover, probably, the disease's consequences will also be resolved swiftly.

Reiki can also be utilized during the healing process. After surgery, patients typically experience pain. The pain a person experiences during the post-surgery recovery period can be alleviated by Reiki's ability to call forth energy, love, and healing. Consequently, the patient will be able to live a richer and more independent life in the coming days.

The experiences of surgical patients who received Reiki would further demonstrate that healing occurs simultaneously with necessary treatment. When most patients would need to transport medical devices such as dextrose and catheters home, those who had Reiki therapy sessions performed on them would leave the hospital with nothing but their clothing attached.

Reiki practitioners and recipients who will soon undergo medical surgery are advised to get at least fifteen full Reiki sessions before the surgery date. If the energy could be transmitted to the accompanying physician, surgeon and nurses, the effect would be even more profound.

Doing so can cut in half the time you need to recover. You will not have to wait six weeks on your recovery bed for the pain to lessen and the wounds to heal, thanks to Reiki. Within three weeks, you should be completely recovered, and you can use the remaining time to continue your self-improvement using Reiki concepts.

Chapter 10: Reiki For Brain Injury.

Reiki is effective on the physical, mental, emotional, and spiritual planes. It employs a precise technique for merging this universal energy with the body's intrinsic healing capabilities.

Reiki is not intended to replace expert medical advice but to complement other therapeutic approaches by promoting profound relaxation. Deep relaxation allows the body to start to mend itself.

Reiki practitioners do not diagnose or prescribe drugs. They instead channel healing energy with their hands. Recipients frequently perceive this energy as warmth or tingling. Many patients fall asleep during therapy sessions, allowing their bodies to relax and heal.

The human energy system, which consists of meridians which are energy channels and chakras, is utilized by Reiki. Also, traditional Chinese Medicine defines twelve major meridians in addition to a governing and functional channel that traverses the body like roadways.

Even though acupuncture was originally seen as purely "alternative," research has revealed a correlation between main acupuncture points and scientifically known nerve pathways and trigger points.

Similarly, chakras- the seven primary energy centers that stretch from the base of the spine to the top of the skull - appear to connect via nerve clusters with endocrine glands whose function or dysfunction results in sensations and physical states connected with the chakras.

The study of meridians and chakras spans millennia, with Western medicine just lately verifying what Chinese and Indian scholars asserted thousands of years ago.

A Reiki practitioner doesn't need to comprehend the human energy system to support it. Through methods most people find baffling, Reiki goes to areas where it is most needed.

In this sense, it functions as what herbalists refer to as an "adaptogen," stimulating weak places while calming overstimulated areas. Considering Reiki's status as "universal life force energy," this makes sense. Nature continually strives towards equilibrium.

A slightly salty mixture is produced when a concentrated saltwater solution is added to fresh water. Yin balances yang. As Reiki passes through the body, rebalancing and natural redistribution of energy occur.

Why It's Effective.

As noted previously, Reiki allows the body to relax sufficiently to repair itself. As a mild, adaptogenic kind of energy, it integrates and reconnects the physical, emotional, mental, and spiritual levels of healing. This is essential for the healing of everyone but especially for TBI survivors.

In some ways, traumatic brain injury is the greatest example of the necessity for multi-level healing. Physical damage affects cognitive and emotional processes. Based on the location of the brain lesion, a person may lose the ability to experience sadness or forget how to perform sequential activities.

Synapses get so disordered that survivors often respond to inquiries "randomly," utilizing whatever connections the brain happens to form at the time. (Mental level) rational thought becomes a struggle.

Depression (emotional level) affects most TBI survivors due in part to neurochemistry and unquestionably to chronic pain and lifestyle loss. Many survivors resort to spiritual pursuits to maintain a good outlook during recovery.

This spiritual inquiry is a natural consequence of an injury that damages a person's sense of self.

What remains if physical harm may erase what we believe we know about ourselves? What is this fundamental Consciousness? Does the cosmos give random blows, or was there a motive for this injury?

If everything happens for a reason, what message might TBI convey? Returning to the concept of chakras, TBI is a problem with the seventh chakra.

The crown chakra is related to the hypothalamus and pineal glands, spirituality, oneness consciousness, and violet and white colors. According to tradition, when an illness or injury affects a certain chakra, the spiritual difficulties associated with that chakra will aid in healing.

The seventh chakra, then, is THE spiritual chakra. Our closest connection to "God Consciousness" or "Universal Love" is the crown of the head. In the same way, the brain influences the entire body, this chakra controls all other chakras.

For most survivors, traumatic brain injury poses obstacles in identifying one's life path, opening to a larger feeling of connection and service, embracing traces of the Divine in everyone and everything, and seeing an underlying order in the cosmos.

Since Reiki addresses all levels of healing, it also assists in balancing the spiritual elements that are so essential to recovery. In contrast to other forms of energy work, Reiki is quite mild.

For instance, Kundalini energy, often known as the human potential that coils at the base of the spine, doesn't manifest as gentle. Kundalini energy is powerful, strong, and forceful, but if aroused too rapidly, it can induce symptoms similar to traumatic brain injury. In contrast, Reiki is always an adaptogen.

It doesn't mandate swift change. Instead, it allows healing to develop and manifest in its own time and manner. Because the seventh chakra is the conclusion of all the other chakras, we may conclude that TBI and other neurological disorders require compassion and respect.

These health conditions are exceedingly complex and changing. Attempting to force recuperation never succeeds, as doing so would demand us to supplant something we do not fully comprehend. Ultimately, TBI gives the most significant opportunity for integration.

Many TBI survivors possess powerful spiritual, artistic, and healing abilities. Therefore, their soul retrieval and recovery have the potential to bring about profound changes in the world. Reiki respects this complex process and fosters a conducive environment for transformation.

Chapter 11: Ways To Improve The Reiki Flow When Someone Is In Pain.

If you find yourself in a scenario where you're in pain or someone else is in agony, and the Reiki doesn't seem to be flowing very well, there are steps you can do. Even when experiencing tremendous pain, there are things You can do to promote the Reiki's flow.

Here are five strategies to strengthen the Reiki flow when treating pain:

1. Remove your ego from the equation! Before each healing session, I always affirm, "I am an open Reiki channel, and my ego has stepped aside." This act as a reminder to allow Reiki to do its work, as I am not the healer.

I am merely a conduit for the energy. The more I engage my ego by thinking such as "I want to get rid of the pain," the less efficient the healing process becomes and the more likely I am to absorb negative energy.

2. Relax and Take a Breath! Focus on your breathing when you are in agony or witnessing the pain of someone you care about. Shallow breathing is not conducive to relaxation. It maintains your panic mode. Observe how much more powerfully the Reiki begins to flow when you calm your breathing and relax.

3. Take a moment to focus and exhale slowly, deep breaths if you injure yourself. When administering Reiki to a person in pain, urge them to focus on breathing and relaxing. Resisting the pain worsens it. Communicate calmly with the person in suffering.

Imagine the anguish leaving the individual, restoring them to their state of health. I imagine the pain's energy being absorbed by the Earth. If you are familiar with Karuna Reiki®, try employing the Kriya and Rama symbol, which helps alleviate pain.

Working knowledge of anatomy facilitates a holistic understanding of the body. If you lack training in anatomy, just do your best. Simply confirm that the body is in a condition of completeness.

4. Have faith that the body can cure itself. Reiki improves and accelerates the healing process. When you allow yourself to rest, knowing that the body has an exceptional capacity for self-repair, the Reiki flows more effectively through You.

Imagine that your hand is a Reiki magnet that draws pain from the body. Have the person you are Reikiing picture your hand taking the pain from their body. This provides them something to concentrate on and accelerates the healing process since their mental state has shifted from one of agony to one of relief.

If you are attuned to the second degree of Reiki, you should not forget the power symbol, CKR.

With this sign, you will feel the Reiki become stronger, particularly after you have relaxed and ceased fretting.

Try to be cool, relaxed, and breathe when using Reiki to alleviate pain. Remind yourself that everything will be well. Try not to think negatively. This only maintains your resistance to the healing process.

Believe that you know what to do. Depending on the circumstances, you may require medical or other expert assistance. In the instance of my daughter, she awoke this morning feeling well.

Chapter 12: Utilizing Reiki To Mend A Heartbreak.

The popular idea regarding heartbreak is that time will cure all wounds. Despite this being undeniably true, there is a technique to expedite the healing process and provide much-needed emotional comfort.

That is the Reiki way! Reiki (pronounced Ray-Key) is healing energy discovered by Dr. Mikao Usui in Japan in the early 20th century and brought to the United States in the 1950s. It is a fantastic approach to speed up the recovery of a broken heart and is now becoming more mainstream as an alternative treatment for healing and well-being.

Reiki is mild and non-invasive, and it has been demonstrated to eliminate energetic blockages in the body, allowing the body to heal more quickly. Reiki can heal ".by carrying good energy across the afflicted portions of the energy field and charging them.

It increases the vibratory level of the energy field within and around the physical body, to which negative ideas and emotions are tied. This enables the negative energy to disintegrate and depart."

Since Reiki operates on both a physical and spiritual level, it provides additional comfort during a breakup. The Reiki practitioner administers Reiki by laying his or her hands on the client and allowing Reiki energy to flow via his or her palm chakras.

The Reiki energy enters the client's body and eliminates any energy obstacles it meets, harmonizing the client's body and spirit. This enables the client to recover from the emotional and spiritual pain created by the breakup.

Many Reiki practitioners can also cleanse and balance their customers' chakras. Having a Reiki practitioner especially clear and balancing one's heart chakra during this delicate period can help one become more loving and kind to oneself and may also allow one to trust and express love more quickly in a future relationship.

Reiki is a simple yet potent holistic technique that everyone can benefit from, especially those who have just suffered a loss. If you believe that Reiki treatments could aid in your healing process, you can locate a local practitioner by conducting an internet search for Reiki practitioners.

However, not all practitioners are the same nor charge the same amount, and simply because a practitioner charges a high fee for therapy doesn't imply that he or she is the finest practitioner.

It is advisable to thoroughly examine all regional practitioners, compare costs and services, and phone a few practitioners to inquire about their practice. Thus, you will have a better sense of each practitioner as an individual and will be able to make your first session with the practitioner with whom you intuitively feel the most comfortable.

In most circumstances, you will feel significantly better physically and mentally after just one session. The most frequent experience of Reiki clients is a sense of intense relaxation and well-being during and after treatment, with more significant therapeutic effects becoming apparent after many sessions.

Reiki is a fantastic method for accelerating emotional recovery, and I highly recommend it to anyone feeling heartache.

Chapter 13: Using A Pendulum During Reiki Healing Treatments.

In many ways, Reiki Masters and practitioners can benefit from using pendulums during Reiki healing sessions. Below, we will explore the three most typical applications of the pendulum in Reiki sessions. However, don't be afraid to think beyond the box! If you allow them, pendulums can help you receive knowledge beyond what your conscious mind knows.

1. Utilize your Reiki pendulum to determine the health of the client's seven primary chakras.

Chakras are the body's energy centers, and the Sanskrit term translates to "wheel." The seven major chakras (root, sacral, solar plexus, heart, throat, third eye, and crown) should rotate clockwise if they are healthy.

Chakras can often become blocked by energy or contain too little or too much energy. Directing the healing Reiki energy towards these unbalanced chakras is an effective method for restoring their equilibrium.

If you hold your Reiki pendulum over each chakra at the start of your session, you may identify which chakras require additional attention and design your Reiki healing session appropriately.

Also, verify the chakras after the Reiki treatment. Observing the client's improvement and how the Reiki healing energy has benefited them is always gratifying.

2. Allow the pendulum to direct your actions throughout a Reiki session (i.e., where to stand, which symbols to give)

To effectively use your pendulum, you must determine its responses before the Reiki therapy. Before you begin your Reiki session, you will want to know how your pendulum responds to "Yes," "No,"

"Maybe," "I don't know," and "Ask later." You may determine the responses of your pendulum by programming and understanding it beforehand.

Assuming you have already configured and comprehended the responses of your Reiki pendulum, utilize it as a valuable instrument, it is during your Reiki sessions by posing queries regarding anything about which you are uncertain. You may be at your client's feet and consult your pendulum to determine if you should remain or move to the person's head.

In addition, a wonderful question is which symbols to employ during the Reiki therapy. Instead of asking questions with your Reiki pendulum, use declarative sentences. For instance, say, "I should place the symbol of forgiveness over the client's heart," and observe the response of your Reiki pendulum. Again, use your imagination!

3. Determine when to administer Reiki and which complementary modalities to employ during the session.

Many Reiki practitioners incorporate crystals, sound healing, aromatherapy, acupressure, and energy work into their practice. Allow your pendulum to assist you in determining not just which complementing instruments to employ and when to arrange sessions to maximize their effectiveness.

Using a Reiki pendulum can be an important tool during treatments, but the beauty of Reiki's healing energy is that it possesses an intelligence of its own. Therefore, there is no wrong method to utilize a pendulum.

Even if you believe you are making a mistake,' which is just a chance to learn, the Reiki healing energy will always get to where it is most needed. So, enjoy using your Reiki pendulum!

Chapter 14: Specify Your Heart's Desire For Your Reiki Practice.

Becoming aware of your heart's intention before beginning your Reiki practice is beneficial. Regardless of your external circumstances and demands, your fundamental motivations for utilizing Reiki will remain the same, even though they may vary and change in tandem with your development. Reiki and your heart's intention will guide you and your practice through the often unexpected changes in your life.

Invoke Reiki and pay attention to your heart's intent. What gifts do you hope to give and receive from your Reiki relationship? What matters the most to you in your deepest heart? Open your heart to the answers you seek. You can listen for your inner direction during both tranquil and hectic periods. Simply activate Reiki and let your everyday life provide the answers.

Invoke Reiki to awaken and link your brain to your heart. The DKM, the Tibetan master symbol, is a potent symbol that can help you become aware of your Reiki heart intention. It facilitates manifestation by balancing giving and receiving. SHK wakes the pure mind, expands the field of possibilities, and unites the divine intellect with the heart.

Request that CKR clean and amplify your voice and connect it to your heart and mind. As you discuss Reiki, you will hear yourself and your definitions. Inviting Reiki to heal your limitations and any worries you may have is an effective way to alleviate them. Request that it reveals your heart's purpose for your Reiki practices.

My heart's purpose is "to promote Reiki worldwide so that children have access to it." My intention has emerged in various ways in my daily life. Yesterday, I instructed my three-year-old grandson Frank on how to administer Reiki to his stubbed toe.

My son and his wife recently asked me to cleanse and bless their new home, and I regularly administer Reiki to my 81-year-old mother. My granddaughter assisted me in teaching him Reiki by blowing Reiki into her hands. This is how Reiki for children manifests in my life.

Simply put, my Reiki business is a manifestation of my heart's intention. More children will be able to benefit from Reiki's healing powers if I can help make it a mainstream profession. This will open the door for more children to train as Reiki practitioners, thereby expanding the Reiki universe even more.

Our work integrating the medical and Reiki communities in Portland, Oregon, has allowed us to see how Reiki's remarkable therapeutic benefits have been recognized in numerous clinics and other medical facilities.

Reiki is something I teach and practice from a spiritual perspective. I've noticed that many of my students and clients turn to me for spiritual body healing for psychological and physical ailments.

As ashamanic practitioner, I use a combination of these two approaches with my clients. I see a lot of clients with spiritual and emotional issues. Because I've experienced the remarkable consequences of their healing, I believe it positively impacts the world.

Every heart's purpose is equal, and all contribute to Reiki's expansion. Reiki can help you hear your voice. Then, follow your heart's intention. It may not always appear to follow your plans. Believe in yourself and keep listening. Continue to ask for Reiki's assistance.

Chapter 15: Reiki Clothing.

Many Reiki healers participated in different trials to determine whether the healing power could be transmitted to others by other means. Due to these millions of experiments, we know many methods for channeling Reiki to others. The most popular approach to obtaining energy is through Reiki-infused clothing.

Reiki clothing is clothing that has been completely imbued with Reiki energy by a skilled Reiki healer. Following a brief meditation, the clothing is imbued with Reiki energy. This outfit imbues the wearer with Reiki energy and envelops the individual in Reiki's potency.

There are many advantages to wearing Reiki clothing, and you will feel the effects when you return to your regular attire. Then you will comprehend the profound transformation that occurred in your mind, body, and spirit.

When is Reiki Clothing acceptable?

Reiki garments containing such powerful energy can be worn at any time. It can be worn during the day while you are most active going about your daily errands; in this way, you will be able to complete your tasks without being fatigued.

Also, you can wear this outfit to bed. This is the period when your body is in the process of recharging, and if you wear Reiki-infused clothing while sleeping, it will considerably improve this process.

You can wear it at festivities or gatherings to improve your shine. Reiki clothing is also great for religious ceremonies; the energy will facilitate a profound connection with the divine.

What types of materials can be utilized to create Reiki Clothing?

Various fabric types are used to create Reiki clothing, but the energy packed into the fabric is important. Cotton, Lycra, cashmere, silk, etc., are used to create Reiki attire. It is believed that silk's characteristics considerably complement Reiki, so silk-made Reiki garments are extremely popular. Other apparel consists of t-shirts, denim jackets, tunics, skirts, slacks, tank tops, and nearly all other fashionable garments.

Advantages of Reiki Clothing.

- Reiki clothing offers various advantages:

- Balances your body's vibrations and invigorates you from the inside out.

- Allows you to experience the full advantages of Reiki energy.

- Allows the body to mend itself.

- Increases your spirit and energy and prevents your energy from becoming depleted.

- Improves your self-assurance and quality of life.

Without performing the real practices, it can now transmit energy to others via Reiki Clothing efficiently. The balanced energy radically transforms your life and your approach to it. Purchase Reiki clothing for yourself and your loved ones. You don't want to lose out on all the marvels this style of clothes can bring into your life.

Chapter 16: Is Reiki Therapy Appropriate For You?

A rising number of hospitals offer Reiki alongside conventional treatments. Reiki practitioners offer treatment in different settings, both privately and in group sessions, where participants learn the Reiki techniques (for themselves and others).

The term "Reiki" is a combination of these two Japanese words: "rei," which means "universal," and "ki," which means "living energy." Its practitioners operate as conduits for primordial awareness (also known as Reiki) while placing their hands lightly on or slightly above the patient.

Reiki originates from Mikao Usui's spiritual teachings in Japan during the early 20th century. It aims to support the individual's healing. According to the National Institutes of Health's Center for

Alternative and Complementary Medicine, it is part of complementary and alternative medicine.

Reiki assists in restoring balance to the physical, emotional, mental, spiritual, and social levels of being. It decreases anxiety and pain and reduces stress. "Beneficiaries often report improved sleep and digestion and an improved sense of well-being.

Other benefits, such as feeling more motivated, less sad, or relieved from the negative effects of drugs, radiation, or chemotherapy, vary from individual to individual. "Reiki A Comprehensive Guide, written by its foremost advocate in the United States, Pamela Miles, states the following.

How Does One Become a Reiki Master?

By attending classes offered by a competent Reiki master, anyone can become a Reiki practitioner. Although it is utilized by nurses, doctors, and other healthcare professionals, it doesn't require a degree or background in healthcare.

The Reiki master gives students Reiki initiation, instruction, and supervised practice during the classes.

During initiation, the student's energy field (the subtle field surrounding and permeating the body) aligns with the limitless primordial consciousness (or energy). "The initiations allow the Reiki student to carry Reiki potential in her hands, which can be activated spontaneously in response to the needs of whoever she touches, herself or another," explains Miles.

There are three levels of Reiki practice: introductory, advanced, and master. The first degree of Reiki prepares the trainee for practice. Second-degree Reiki training prepares the practitioner to provide Reiki treatment at a distance. A Reiki practitioner who becomes a Reiki master is prepared to instruct.

Is Reiki Safe?

Reiki has no negative side effects. "It can only benefit, never harm," Miles asserts. There is no "overdose" of Reiki.

In contrast to energy healing techniques such as Therapeutic Touch and Healing Touch, in which practitioners direct energy and repair imbalances based on assessment results, Reiki practitioners merely act as conduits for Reiki.

The recipient's specific needs determine the flow and application of Reiki. The practitioner has no cognitive control or direction over the energy.

How Should One Select a Reiki Practitioner?

Education and experience are more significant than the sort of practitioner, according to Miles. A first-degree Reiki practitioner may have more direct Reiki therapeutic experience than a second-degree Reiki practitioner or even a Reiki master.

Suggestions for locating a practitioner:

- Request a reference from your doctor, nurse, or other health professional.

- Check with practitioners of holistic, complementary, or integrative medicine. They may provide the service themselves or know a competent practitioner.

- Simply request Reiki while in the hospital.

- Ask your buddies. You could be shocked to discover that one of them offers Reiki or knows someone who does.

- Consult the Reiki Alliance, an organization of Reiki Masters that provides referrals and information on Reiki.

Once you have identified practitioners, describe your needs to them. Inquire about their training and experience practicing Reiki. Determine who they are and why they are practicing Reiki. Determine their pricing, billing, and cancellation policies. Not only is this information useful, but it also provides insight into the individual.

Choose a practitioner who suits your needs and with whom you are comfortable.

Reiki treatment provides spiritual healing. Your particular demands influence Reiki's flow and utilization.

Choosing a Reiki practitioner based on their experience and your needs is more crucial than the type of practitioner (first degree, second degree, or master's).

Reiki therapy should not be used as a substitute for visiting a healthcare provider for serious health issues; nonetheless, many patients benefit from combining Reiki with medical procedures and treatments. Reiki requires neither your faith nor your willingness to experience it.

Chapter 17: How Reiki Therapy Can Benefit Seniors.

As we age, our bodies struggle to perform routine tasks, and life is not always as enjoyable as we would like. In varying degrees, pains and aches in our muscles and joints, slow-healing wounds, and unsightly bruises hinder the pleasure of our old age.

However, it shouldn't have to be this way. These irritating, bothersome discomforts can be decreased, diminished, and in many cases eliminated with regular Reiki sessions.

Old and young people worldwide have benefited from Reiki to treat stress, painful injuries, diseases, and physical, emotional, and mental ailments. Unfortunately, not all elders are aware of the benefits of Reiki.

Reiki is a peaceful, ancient, hands-on therapy that links us to the universal life force energy that science affirms encompasses every person and living thing. A Reiki practitioner isn't a healer in the traditional sense but is taught to channel this energy to needy individuals through their hands.

Most seniors only utilize conventional medication. Reiki is not a substitute for this medication. As a complementary treatment, it works with doctors and other medical professionals. Reiki is compassionate, delicate, and manual. It is intended primarily to decrease stress and clear energy blockages from the body.

After all, we are mainly energy; like other systems, we occasionally "blow up." This is regarded as an "energetic blockage" in Reiki, as it prevents the usual flow of energy into and out of our bodies.

Reiki Therapeutic Touch.

People of all ages are experiencing and benefiting from the Reiki touch (or non-contact, as

Reiki is equally beneficial when the practitioner's hands are placed a few inches above the body as when they are placed directly on the body) with increasing frequency. Usually, one session is sufficient to begin to feel the difference.

Even those who have undergone chemotherapy or major surgery often notice a reduction in recovery time and a reduction in discomfort after receiving Reiki treatment. People who are sensitive to the touch of others owing to neurological or other illnesses might also benefit from Reiki because it is equally effective without physical contact.

Reiki produces an atmosphere that promotes relaxation through quiet music, dim lighting, and a cozy setting. This is very enticing to seniors. Falling asleep during a session is natural and has no negative impact on the outcome. If it helps you relax and accept the treatment, take a nap.

Most seniors who receive Reiki treatments report instant symptom improvement. In certain cases, it may take many days to manifest. Similar to how medicine doesn't function the same for everyone, a small minority of patients report no difference. However, family and friends often report observing favorable physical or mental changes.

Reiki is most effective when the recipient believes in the efficacy of energy healing. Understanding how Reiki works and having faith in its curative potential goes a long way toward acceptance and receiving benefits from the Reiki practitioner's energy transfer.

Reiki is sometimes viewed with skepticism by seniors because it is a new-age treatment rather than the conventional methods they are accustomed to. Consequently, an initial shorter session may be recommended. This would be followed by additional Reiki education through reading about how Reiki has helped others, which would eventually lead to a one-hour treatment.

Reiki, Elderly People, and Everyday Life.

Most seniors I know suffer from joint and muscular stiffness, aches, pains, circulation issues, and neurological diseases. Reiki can often alleviate these symptoms and help seniors enjoy their golden years more.

Reiki is typically readily accepted by the elderly since it delivers the desired relief. It helps alleviate their pain and suffering and improves their ability to move their muscles and joints without any fear of pain, assisting with typical occurrences such as falls.

Remember a time as a child when you were injured? The first thing your mother did was place her hand on the injured spot, and she probably also kissed it to make it feel better. Such is Reiki! As stated previously, Reiki assists most individuals, especially the elderly, to recover from surgery and injuries more quickly.

Reiki treatment can also alleviate various common issues among seniors, such as respiratory issues and decreased energy and activity levels. Reiki can typically bring about a general improvement in cognitive function. Dry, itchy skin is a major aggravation for many senior citizens. This may result from different sources. Reiki might also bring relief to this situation.

Another common senior ailment that Reiki can treat is insomnia. Reiki is so calming and relaxing that, with some instruction in Reiki self-healing, insomniacs can learn how to get a restful night's sleep every night.

Too many senior citizens cannot enjoy their retirement due to physical or mental health issues, such as depression, memory loss, forgetfulness, Alzheimer's disease, or dementia. Seniors have a better chance of experiencing greater life satisfaction with Reiki care.

Dementia is a devastating disease that robs individuals of their memories, and in the late stages, they often do not even know their own families. Sad! However, Reiki can often reach these dementia patients through its gentle treatment.

According to a research study by the University of California, Los Angeles (UCLA), Reiki has the power to alleviate stress, anxiety, and depression, all of which influence dementia patients. Reiki has made such amazing inroads into Western medicine that it is currently available in approximately 900 hospitals in the United States.

Reiki improves the quality of life for the elderly.

Seniors often have to deal with memory loss, diminished ability to function normally, muscle aches, joint and chronic pain, disabilities, uncomfortable and embarrassing disorders such as incontinence or the inability to do things for themselves, constant medical visits, morning and evening meditations and a multitude of other issues that detract from the enjoyment of what are supposed to be their happy retirement years.

Our senior adults are fortunate that Reiki is accessible to assist in alleviating their aches and bring some relaxation and delight into their life. Reiki may make a difference by reducing their degree of pain, suffering, and illness while boosting their energy flow and, consequently, their ability to perform better, restoring their enjoyment of life and enhancing their health, safety, and well-being.

Reiki as a Pain Reliever.

A study undertaken by the US government determined that Reiki might assist minimize discomfort and the need for medicines in patients undergoing medical procedures.

Reiki as an Addition to Conventional Medicine.

Reiki doesn't substitute conventional treatment or medical attention. It is a complementary therapy and collaborates with physicians and other healthcare professionals. It has been demonstrated to positively benefit patients, accelerate the healing process, and expedite their return to full health. Occasionally, Reiki is effective when other treatments fail.

Reiki and Major Conditions.

Reiki is also proving effective in delivering pain treatment to patients with serious illnesses, such as those undergoing heart surgery and cancer. Chemotherapy patients who receive Reiki treatment in addition to their typical recuperation often notice a reduction in discomfort.

The medical community has started realizing the benefits of Reiki therapy for people in general, especially the elderly. As stated previously, Reiki therapy is now offered in 900 hospitals in the United States.

It is expanding rapidly as more and more people realize how effective Reiki can be in treating different diseases and disorders. Why? Because Reiki has proven to be an effective complement or auxiliary to conventional medical treatment. Reiki is effective, and it can help you.

Chapter 18: FAQs About Reiki.

What are Reiki and Seichem?

Reiki and Seichem are therapeutic techniques that transmit energy into the body through the practitioner's hands. Although Reiki and Seichem are more commonly linked with emotional and mental healing than physical problems, the popular belief is that to be well on the exterior, one must also be healthy on the inside, and based on this premise, both can heal physical ailments and emotional ones.

Where does Reiki come from?

Reiki is a time-honored Asian practice for both the treatment of present diseases and the prevention of future illnesses. Reiki, believed to have originated in Japan, has also been associated with certain disciplines of traditional Chinese medicine.

The actual history of Reiki is partially obscured by myth, and the truth may never be fully revealed. According to the information now accessible, Dr. Mikao Usui invented Reiki after a 21-day fast and meditation practice on Mount Kurama, one of many sacred mountains in Japan, where he was alone. This information is only recently available outside of Japan, and its integrity cannot be confirmed.

Unquestionably, Mrs. Hawayo Takata from Hawaii was the first to introduce the Usui system of natural medicine to the western world. Mrs. Takata was effectively treated Dr. Hayashi for a chronic illness at his Reiki clinic in Tokyo while visiting relatives in Japan. Dr. Hayashi attuned her to Reiki, after which she could practice Reiki, and introduced her to other practitioners.

How does Reiki work?

Reiki is one of some holistic therapies centered on various points of the body, similar to acupuncture and reflexology. All these holistic, energy-based treatments are based on the body's natural "chakras" and energy fields or auras, are rooted in ancient Asian philosophies, and are extremely similar to one another.

In contrast to reflexology, which includes rubbing or applying pressure to specific energy points, and acupuncture, which requires inserting needles into various locations, Reiki doesn't necessarily require the practitioner to touch the patient.

By placing the hands lightly on or just above a sequence of spots on the recipient's body, energy is channeled to the body's acupuncture points. The energy goes via the practitioner and directly into the recipient's body via the acupuncture points but isn't generated by the practitioner and doesn't exhaust his or her energy reserves.

Even skilled practitioners can deliver treatment remotely, although this is a very complex technique that novice practitioners should not attempt.

Who can administer and/or receive Reiki?

Learning Reiki doesn't involve any unique skills or extensive research. You can learn to administer Reiki treatments to yourself, loved ones, animals, and plants. Some individuals even employ Reiki on appliances.

It stands to reason that a healing method that utilizes pure energy will mend or cure inefficiencies in the workings of such organisms and objects, given that everything in the universe operates by utilizing some type of energy.

Everyone has the latent ability to channel specialized healing energy, but this power must be activated through attunement. Regardless of age or other considerations, anyone can become attuned and learn how to channel Reiki successfully.

After receiving attunement from an experienced Reiki master, you can practice Reiki and share its benefits with others in addition to treating yourself. Reiki may treat, revitalize and heal the practitioner and the patient.

What specific benefits does Reiki offer?

Illness occurs when the body, mind, and spirit are out of balance. Reiki can help ease pain and illness's physical, emotional, mental, and spiritual suffering. Essentially, this suggests that Reiki is capable of healing.

Emotional disorders and physical diseases are both caused by disruptions in the personal energy field, and genuine health can only be reached by returning the complete being to harmony and balance with itself, the Earth, and the universe. Reiki is among the most effective methods for restoring this equilibrium and harmony.

Reiki can be utilized daily, unlike conventional western medicine, which is only used for the treatment of certain conditions during suffering and under the supervision of a physician.

Reiki assists the recovery of people undergoing medical treatment but can also be utilized for illness prevention. As sickness is produced by imbalance, maintaining constant equilibrium can only be beneficial, minimizing the likelihood of being unwell.

Many individuals find the Reiki treatment so enjoyable that they indulge in frequent sessions as a refreshing and soothing treat for themselves, similar to how they may receive a massage, facial, guided visualization session, or mud bath.

What is the purpose of Reiki?

Reiki promotes relaxation and reduces stress by releasing blocked energy from the body and mind. Natural energy has an inbuilt intelligence. Therefore, it doesn't matter where on the body the therapy is directed; it will spontaneously re-direct itself and go to wherever it is needed, assisting in eliminating toxins from the body. Reiki is also effective on plants, animals, machines, and other inanimate objects.

Reiki is a technique that empowers and enables us to become whole in every manner. We initiate our recovery by acting on our desire to be healthy and whole. Without the desire to be healthy, we cannot become healthy.

When Reiki is provided, the flow of energy via the aura and into the actual body is increased. Reiki energy helps to harmonize or bring into balance the physical, emotional, mental, and spiritual components that make up the entirety of the individual.

Reiki dissolves emotional barriers, trauma, and energy blocks in other aspects of 'you,' ensuring that you remain physically and emotionally balanced.

Does any evidence exist that proves Reiki works?

Scientists and medical doctors are hesitant to acknowledge the efficacy of energy healing treatments. However, many studies have demonstrated a rapid and significant improvement in health following different energy therapies. Aura photos have also revealed significant alterations before and during Reiki treatments.

This is not a guarantee that any sickness will be alleviated by a single or many Reiki treatments. Reiki should not be used as a substitute for expert medical treatment, especially in the case of serious illness.

However, Reiki appears to improve the effects of medical treatment when used in conjunction with it and the body's innate ability to heal. Patients receiving both medical and Reiki treatments appear to recover more swiftly and completely.

The essential premise of Reiki is that it cannot cause harm and cannot be utilized for harmful purposes; hence, there is no danger in doing something that may benefit one's healing.

While the use of Reiki to heal illness and injury may be contentious, its use as a therapy for relaxation and stress reduction is becoming increasingly acknowledged and popular. Reiki improves other bodywork, healing procedures, athletic performance, and spiritual development.

Conclusion.

There are other healers today, including medical healers, auric healers, clairvoyants, and psychics, but very few have the track record that Reiki Masters have today. Reiki originated in Japan around 1922; it is an alternative form of medicine using a form of hands-on treatment.

Reiki is a healing therapy that, similar to acupuncture, configures the body's energetic systems through transferring universal energy through the hands. This essay will enlighten you on Reiki symbols and why they are crucial for Reiki Masters today.

Reiki was created in Japan by Mikao Usui, a Buddhist who was a very skilled hands-on healer. Although this is considered an oriental medicine, anyone attuned to the Reiki symbols by a Reiki Master can access the same healing power.

Understanding that healing is about achieving perfect balance, the energy that pours from your hands simply restores a person's equilibrium. Since science has demonstrated that energy and matter are inextricably interrelated, changing the energy flow within a person can likewise result in a physical alteration.

There are two regularly performed varieties of Reiki. The first is known as traditional Japanese Reiki. The latter is known as Western Reiki. Traditional Reiki is more intuitive, with the healer placing his or her hands in spots where he or she believes the energy should flow.

Western Reiki focuses on a highly systematic method of laying one's hands on a person's body to transform. Both have three levels: a first, a second, and a level known as a master teacher. You can only acquire the attenuation of all three levels and become a Reiki Master from a master instructor.

Reiki can aid in individuals' healing since it can tap into Ki. This is also referred to as Chi in China and by many other names in cultures around the world. In essence, you are tapping into the energy from whence all things originated, the spirit of the cosmos.

Doing so can detach yourself from the circumstance and temporarily pause the internal debate or your perspective of the environment to allow the energy to flow through you.

The Reiki symbols might assist you in gaining access to the healing forces of the universe. You will have a higher chance of becoming a more skilled healer if you are attuned to a Reiki Master who utilizes the symbols at all three levels.

The correct reply is both yes and no. Healing may not develop if a person is not healed by a Reiki Master or by anyone running energy due to the energetic frequencies of both the healer and the person. It works for everyone, but depending on the circumstances, it might not.

It is also imperative to understand that the universe operates on its timetable and that when a person's time arrives, it is their time to depart. We can only try our best to give them the best possible chance of recovering from their illness or injuries, but this doesn't mean Reiki is ineffective if our efforts fail.

In the same way that doctors must adhere to particular guidelines that give them the best possible opportunity of saving a patient's life, they are not always successful. Therefore, attempting to heal someone with Reiki doesn't decrease its power to aid in healing.

In conclusion, to become a Reiki Master, you must have a strong understanding of Reiki symbols. If you can run energy spontaneously or if your hands grow heated, and if you have impacted good change in others through hands-on healing or distance healing, learning the Reiki symbols and becoming a Reiki Master can make you a greater healer.

I hope this information should motivate you to discover more about Reiki and all the great effects it can have not just on the people you care about but also on your own life.

Thanks for reading

This book is part of an ongoing collection called "Why Alternative Medicine Works"

1. Why Yoga Works
2. Why Chakra Works
3. Why Massage Therapy Works
4. Why Reflexology Works
5. Why Acupuncture Works
6. Why Reiki Works
7. Why Meditation Works
8. Why Hypnosis Works
9. Why Colon Cleansing Works
10. Why Crystal Healing Works
11. Why NLP (Neuro Linguistic Programming) Works
12. Why Energy Healing Works
13. Why Foot Detoxing Works
14. Why Singing Bowls Works.

Other Series by Sherry Lee

"Using Sage and Smudging"

1. Learning About Sage and Smudging
2. Sage and Smudging for Love

3. Sage and Smudging for Health and Healing
4. Sage and Smudging for Wealth and Abundance
5. Sage and Smudging for Spiritual Cleansing
6. Sage and Smudging for Negativity.

"Learning About Crystals"

1. Crystals for Love
2. Crystals for Health
3. Crystals for Wealth
4. Crystals for Spiritual Cleansing
5. Crystals for Removing Negativity.

"What Every Newlywed Should Know and Discuss Before Marriage."

1. Newlywed Communication on Money
2. Newlywed Communication on In-laws
3. Newlywed Communication about Children.
4. Newlywed Communication on Religion.
5. Newlywed Communication on Friends.
6. Newlywed Communication on Retirement.
7. Newlywed Communication on Sex.
8. Newlywed Communication on Boundaries.

9. Newlywed Communication on Roles and Responsibilities.

"Health is Wealth."

1. Health is Wealth
2. Positivity is Wealth
3. Emotions is Wealth.
4. Social Health is Wealth.
5. Happiness is Wealth.
6. Fitness is Wealth.
7. Meditating is Wealth.
8. Communication is Wealth.
9. Mental Health is Wealth.
10. Gratitude is Wealth.

"Personal Development Collection."

1. Manifesting for Beginners
2. Crystals for Beginners
3. How to Manifest More Money into your Life.
4. How to work from home more effectively.
5. How to Accomplish more in Less Time.
6. How to End Procrastination.
7. Learning to Praise and acknowledge your Accomplishments.
8. How to Become your Own Driving Force.

9. Creating a Confident Persona.

10. How to Meditate.

11. How to Set Affirmations.

12. How to Set and Achieve your Goals.

13. Achieving Your Fitness Goals.

14. Achieving Your Weight Loss Goals.

15. How to Create an Effective Vision Board.

Other Books By Sherry Lee:

- **Repeating Angel Numbers**
- **Most Popular Archangels.**

Author Bio

Sherry Lee. Sherry enjoys reading personal development books, so she decided to write about something she is passionate about. More books will come in this collection, so follow her on Amazon for more books.

Thank you for your purchase of this book.

I honestly do appreciate it and appreciate you, my excellent customer.

God Bless You.

Sherry Lee.

Made in the USA
Monee, IL
12 November 2022

17642507R00066